SIXTY FI

The

RICHARD C. GANNON

Story

By

ROSEZELLE BOGGS-QUALLS

Rosezelle Boggs-Qualls

Edited by Barbara Brunk
Cuyahoga Falls, Ohio

To the best of the author's knowledge, this is a true story. It is based on personal interviews with Richard C. Gannon and his family, and on extensive research involving innumerable mementoes consisting of photographs, letters, national newspaper and magazine articles, and historical data written and preserved by Richard's mother, Mary Elizabeth Moon, and his sister, Barbara Brunk.

An Ascended Ideas original

Ascended Ideas ePublishing
PO Box 120
Coldiron, KY 40819
http://www.ascendedideas.com

ISBN: 13: 978-0-9795103-4-2 10: 0-9795103-4-1

Cover by Judy A Mason

Printed in the United States of America

Sixty Five Roses: The Richard C. Gannon Story

I have dedicated this book:

To my children, Daniel, Ginger, Mitchell, Barbara and Richard.

To Life Banc and the transplant surgeons at University Hospitals
of Cleveland who performed the
surgeries on my son.

And,

Special thanks to Ann Heck of Redding, California, for donating
her son's organs in 1998, and
to the other loving families who donated their
loved ones' organs in 1991 so that
my son could live.

God Bless.

Dedication by

Mary Elizabeth Moon

For their kind encouragement, and
assistance, I extend my appreciation
to relatives and friends:

Chuck Bianchi, Baxter, Kentucky
Reverend Titus Boggs, Laurel Mission, Big Laurel, Kentucky
Bela Bognar, PhD, Wright State University, Dayton, Ohio
Carl Brun, PhD, Chair, Social Work Department,
        Wright State University, Dayton, Ohio
Barbara Brunk. Cuyahoga Falls, Ohio
Timothy Campbell, Cawood, Kentucky
Terri Campbell, Cawood, Kentucky
Richard C. Gannon, Akron, Ohio
Judie Golden, Stow, Ohio
Judith Victoria Hensley, Loyall, Kentucky
Anne Rose Greene, Richmond, Indiana
Curtis and Nancy Greene, Richmond, Indiana
Reverend Doctor Daryl C. Greene, Richmond, Indiana
Emily Street-Hensel, Navarre, Ohio
Donna Jones, Miamisburg, Ohio
Bobbie Maggard, Cumberland, Kentucky
Gayle Warstler-Miller, Navarre, Ohio
Mary Moon, Akron, Ohio
Mary Frances Young-Qualls, Cawood, Kentucky
Rebecca L. Qualls, Doylestown, Ohio
Thomas S. Qualls, North Canton, Ohio
Vickie Qualls, Mary Alice, Kentucky
William A. (Buck) Qualls, Cawood, Kentucky
Leroy and Kathy Schindler, New Lebanon, Ohio
Karen Wilson-Zenner, Akron, Ohio

With sincere thanks,

Rosezelle Boggs-Qualls

ABOUT THE AUTHOR

From the rugged mountains of Southeastern Kentucky comes one of the twenty first century's most powerful writers. Her written word will both educate and entertain you.

Rosezelle Boggs-Qualls grew up in Sunshine, a small coal mining village just south of Harlan, Kentucky. A born tomboy, she spent her days exploring the trails, streams, caves and abandoned mines of the Cumberland, Big Black and the Pine Mountains. For High School, Rosezelle attended the Pine Mountain Settlement School, Pine Mountain, Kentucky. In spite of a serious hearing impairment, she graduated from high school at age 16. In 1946 she met and married William (Buck) Qualls. Her husband is totally deaf.

When they were first married they lived in Cawood, Kentucky. However in 1947, Harlan was a depressed area and in order to find employment they were forced to leave the mountains that they loved and moved to Dayton, Ohio.

Rosezelle earned a Bachelor of Science Degree in Social Work at Wright State University, Dayton, Ohio. Her graduate work in Applied Behavioral Science was also at Wright State. For more than 35 years she was employed as a social work administrator in the Child Welfare field in both the Dayton and Akron, Ohio areas. After her retirement in 2004, she and Buck came back home to relocate in Harlan and now live in Cawood, Kentucky. They have one son, Tom, three grandchildren, one rescued dog, and eight rescued cats.

In 2003 Rosezelle was given the prestigious Wright State Social Worker of the Year Award, and the Wright State College of Liberal Arts Most Outstanding Alumna Award.

Also, Rosezelle served a six year appointment to The Ohio Governor's Council on People with Disabilities 1998-2004. She is serving her first appointed term to the Kentucky Governor's Statewide Independent Living council (SILC) for people with disabilities and she is now serving her second term as Board Chairperson for the Pathfinders for Independent Living Agency whose offices are in Harlan.

In 2007 she organized and is now serving her second term as President of the Harlan Writers' Guild.

BOOKS BY ROSEZELLE BOGGS-QUALLS

"SIXTY FIVE ROSES: THE RICHARD C. GANNON STORY

This is an inspirational true story. Documented by his family, it chronicles the life of Akron, Ohio native Richard C. Gannon. Born in 1952 with **Cystic Fibrosis** and a life expectancy of age 11, he becomes financially independent, operates his own business, and is an award winning hunter, and fisherman.

'**Sixty Five Roses: The Richard C. Gannon Story**" pays tribute to the medical skills of his doctors, the commitment of Life Banc, the loving families of organ donors, and tells how a man's courage, faith in God, the awesome power of prayer, and his family's love and support enabled him to overcome incredible life threatening challenges. He is the first person in Ohio to successfully receive a triple-organ transplant in one surgery. (a liver, kidney, and pancreas) The sixteen-hour surgery was performed in January, 1991, at the University Hospitals of Cleveland and made medical history around the world.

"WALKING FREE: THE NELLIE ZIMMERMAN STORY"

The author, together with legally blind Reverend Doctor Daryl C. Greene, Richmond, Indiana, wrote an inspirational landmark book about a totally deaf and totally blind lady from Massillon, Ohio titled "Walking Free: The Nellie Zimmerman Story."

Nellie had a deep abiding faith in God. Abandoned by her family, she was locked up in a mental hospital only because no one could communicate with her. After 19 years of silence, at age 71, Nellie was released. Then she went to college, lectured all over northeast Ohio, and became an award winning life skills teacher of deaf/blind teenage boys!

"THE BLACK HEART BOOK" (AND ITS SEQUEL)

This is an **on-going** inspirational true story about the Southeastern Kentucky Mountains and the author's great grandfather, Alex Turner and her grandmother, Judy Turner Smith. "**The Black Heart Book**" is about terrible sin and redemption, and chronicles events that affected the Turner family from 1898 on into the 1900's.

"OUR CAT FAMILY"

This is a true story about eight rescued cats and how their individual stories intermingle with the events that impacted the lives of their human family.

SIXTY FIVE ROSES: THE RICHARD C. GANNON STORY
By
Rosezelle Boggs-Qualls

CONTENTS

SIXTY FIVE ROSES: THE RICHARD C. GANNON STORY
By
Rosezelle Boggs-Qualls

PHOTOGRAPHS
(Provided by Richard Gannon, Barbara Brunk, and Mary Moon)

PROLOGUE

This true story is about a man of great courage, and it pays a fitting tribute to the indomitable human spirit. The chronicling of Richard's life story reveals how he and his family struggled to successfully overcome his constant life-threatening health challenges. For his ability to have a consistently enriched quality of life, Richard credits the awesome professional skills and commitment to his medical needs by his doctors, the strength he draws from his family through their strong faith in God, the awesome power of prayer, and an abiding love.

"SIXTY FIVE ROSES: THE RICHARD C. GANNON STORY" is a true story as related to the author by Richard's mother, Mary Elizabeth Moon, his sister, Barbara Brunk, and by Richard C. Gannon, himself. His story is well documented by innumerable family mementoes consisting of photographs and national newspaper and magazine articles.

The title for Richard's story comes from an interview the author had with his mother, Mary Moon. She related that in 1957 when Richard was five years old she overheard him explaining to a playmate why he was sick so much. "He couldn't pronounce cystic fibrosis, so he did the best he could. He told his playmate that he was sick and had to take a whole lot of pills everyday because he had **sixty five roses**."

In the late fifties and through the sixties, several support groups for the families and victims struggling with cystic fibrosis in Northeast Ohio adopted Richard's name for his disease and called themselves the Sixty Five Roses Support Groups.

Cystic fibrosis in a newborn child is a medical diagnosis so dreadful that it strikes fear in the hearts of the afflicted child's loved ones.

In 2003, according to the Cystic Fibrosis Foundation, some 30,000 Americans have CF, about twelve million people are CF carriers, and each year there are twenty-five hundred babies born with CF.

Cystic fibrosis is the most commonly known fatal inherited disease. CF causes the body to produce thick sticky mucus mostly in the lungs and throughout the respiratory system. It also affects the pancreas, which causes major digestive problems.

CF results from the inheritance of a defective autosomal recessive gene. A person who has only one copy of the gene is a "CF carrier." When two CF carriers become the father and mother of a child, there is a twenty-five percent chance the baby will be born with cystic fibrosis. A person born with CF has inherited the gene from both parents.

Cystic fibrosis has far reaching affects on the human body. CF alters the mucus secretions of the epithelial cells that make up the outside layer of tissue that lines all of the open surfaces of the body, including the tunnels and cavities in the lungs, urinary tract, liver, colon, and reproductive tract. The heavy, thick, sticky mucus clogs the airways to the lungs, making them vulnerable to continual infection. The mucus blocks the pancreatic juices flowing through the pancreas and impedes both digestion and absorption of vital nutrients. This leads to serious nutritional deficiencies and life threatening intestinal complications.

In recent years there have been many dramatic medical improvements in the treatment and longevity of CF patients. A baby born with CF prior to 1940 had a life expectancy of about two years. A baby born today with CF has a life expectancy of about thirty years.

Richard Cummins Gannon was born on September 19, 1952, the youngest of four children. He has one brother, two sisters, and a half brother. Each of his parents unknowingly carried the defective autosomal recessive gene. He is the only child in their family to be diagnosed with cystic fibrosis. By being born in 1952, Richard had a life expectancy of less than twelve years.

However, Richard is a survivor! To the author's knowledge, in January, 2007, he is one of the oldest living persons diagnosed with cystic fibrosis as an infant. With the ever progression of modern medicine, his own constant faith in God, and the love, prayers, and support of his family and friends, he courageously persevered through many overpowering life challenges.

Richard is the first known person to successfully undergo a triple-organ transplant. At University Hospitals of Cleveland, he received a new liver, kidney and pancreas. The surgery took sixteen hours and the doctors who performed the miraculous multiple organ transplant surgery made medical news around the world!

Chapter 1
A BLESSED CHILD

On September 19, 1952, Mary and Manuel Gannon were blessed with a beautiful baby boy. They named him Richard Cummins Gannon, after his paternal grandfather. At first, all seemed to be fine for both mother and baby. However, on that first day, his mother was concerned because her baby's stomach was not retaining his formula. As soon as he managed to take just two ounces from his bottle, he stopped sucking and his little face and cry showed he was in distress. Then, within a few minutes the formula came back up.

Finally, that long first day came to a close. When the night nurse brought little Richard to his mother, Mary said, "I'm not sure what's wrong, but will you please tell the doctor that my baby isn't retaining anything he takes of his formula?"

"I wouldn't worry just yet," the nurse replied, "some babies are born with diarrhea."

"No," Mary said, "It isn't diarrhea. I know it's more than that. Will you please inform the doctor that something's wrong, seriously wrong? I believe he needs to know this right away!"

Despite her misgivings, and anxious questioning of the hospital's resident pediatrician, Mary received no viable answers and she and her baby boy were dismissed on schedule from Akron City Hospital.

Mary called their pediatrician, Doctor Lewis Walker, the next morning and made an appointment for that afternoon. After a thorough examination by Dr. Walker, he told the anxious parents, "In order to be sure of my diagnosis, I want you to take

Richard to Babies' and Children's Hospital in Cleveland. I'll call now and make an appointment for you."

Their appointment was on the very next day at Cleveland Children's Hospital and was with a lady whose name was Doctor Startzman, a staff pediatrician. Both Mary and Manuel were reassured by the doctor. "Your baby is not in any immediate danger; however, I'll need to run laboratory tests and to have enough time to conduct some research before I'll be able to identify your son's digestive problem. We'll schedule his blood work and x-rays in our lab today before you leave the hospital. I'll make a follow-up appointment for you to return in two days."

On their second trip, Dr, Startzman greeted them and then invited them into her office. "I don't have good news about your son. After running the tests and assessing the results, I've found the answer to his condition. Your son has a rare genetic disease called cystic fibrosis.

This is a disease of the lungs and pancreas. With this condition there is a constant presence of thick sticky mucus that clogs the lungs and respiratory system. It also clogs the pancreas and blocks the flow of the digestive juice tripsen. Digestive juices allow food to digest and for the absorption of vital nutrients for the body. It's critical to your son's survival that we find the right formula for him. One that will allow him to take his bottle, digest and retain the nutrients in his food."

The two parents sat in stunned silence while Dr. Startzman explained her diagnosis. Finally, Mary recovered enough to ask the questions uppermost in her mind. "Will he be all right? Is the disease treatable? What do we need to do? What is cystic fibrosis, and how did he get it?"

Dr. Startzman replied, in great detail. "I'll try to answer the questions you have now. I know you'll have many more questions later. I'll work with Dr. Walker, your pediatrician in Akron, and with you to see that your son receives the medical care he needs. Yes, the disease is treatable. Both Dr. Walker and I will give you instructions for his care at home. You'll know what to do, and will be able to call either of us at anytime with any questions or concerns about your son's care."

Dr. Startzman continued to talk with the anxious parents in a soothing, compassionate voice. "Cystic fibrosis was brought over to the United States by three European brothers in 1610. My research indicates that in order for a child to be born with this genetic disease, both parents must carry the gene. You are both carriers. But, you are only carriers. Neither of you have the disease yourself, but you have unknowingly passed it on to your baby boy."

After she recovered from the initial feeling of grief and shock, Mary paid close attention to the instructions and training she received that day from Dr. Startzman. With baby Richard at home she would be his primary caregiver. The doctor said that he would have to be given more than thirty different medications.

The ever present danger to their baby was Richard's susceptibility to pneumonia. The doctor said "Pneumonia will always be life threatening for your son and when you see the very first sign of pneumonia developing in baby Richard, call your family doctor and rush him to the hospital for early treatment."

Mary had an older son named Daniel, who was by her first husband. He was almost five years older than the oldest of Mary's and Manuel's other four children: Ginger, Mitchell, Barbara and baby Richard. Their children had been born just about a year apart. Ginger, their oldest child was almost five years old.

Richard's brothers and sisters were too young to understand the seriousness of their baby brother's illness. Daniel and Ginger listened solemnly as Mary explained to them, "Little Richard is going to require special medical care. I'll have to depend on you, Daniel, and Ginger, to help me with some of the house work. I'll have to depend on you to help me to take care of Mitchell and Barbara. I'll have to attend to your baby brother the greater part of my time. Will you both help me?"

Daniel's and Ginger's eyes grew huge as they solemnly nodded, "Yes."

Every morning Mary began the day with a prayer. She thanked God that Richard's doctors were always available, both day and night, to answer her questions and address her concerns.

It was to Dr. Walker that she turned most often. Uppermost in her prayers was that God would lead her to find the right formula that would allow Richard's digestive system to tolerate his food and retain the nutrients he so desperately needed. Mary tried every known baby formula on the market without success. She even tried goat's milk! Nothing was working. Richard kept losing weight and she was desperate.

After what seemed to be endless days, she finally found a newly marketed brand of baby formula called Vita-Lak. This formula contained the vitamins and minerals he needed, but was minus the high fat content of the others. She fervently prayed, "Please, dear Lord, let this formula work for my baby."

As soon as he was given his first bottle of the Vita-Lak formula, Richard greedily finished six ounces of the milk and peacefully fell asleep. Over the next two days, Mary watched in amazement as he quickly finished each bottle that she gave him. As she continued to pray that the new formula would be tolerated by his digestive system, she could only watch and wait.

The first day, Richard seemed frantic as he took each bottle of the new formula. By his actions anyone could tell that he was literally starved for the nourishment. By the end of the second day, it was apparent to Mary that her baby was tolerating Vita-Lak.

Mary couldn't help it. She was in tears. Her tears were tears of joy as she exclaimed, "Oh, praise be to God! Our long search is over! God is with us. My baby is going to be all right now. Thank you, dear Lord Jesus, my prayers have been answered!"

With anxious eyes, Mary prayerfully watched his daily progress and soulfully rejoiced as Richard's thin little body began to put on weight. After a few days, with the warm and comforting secure feeling that came from finally having plentiful nourishment, Richard stopped his frantic greediness. He cooed as he took his bottle and made the normal baby noises that his mother desperately wanted to hear.

Daniel and Ginger were true to their promise to help their mother with the housework and the care of their younger brother and sister. Daniel was in school, but Ginger was too young to go to school and was still at home with her mother. She had a special bond with her brothers and sister. Barbara, the youngest, showed a special love for her baby brother and was a great help to her mother by just sitting by his crib, holding his hand and cooing to him in baby talk.

For the next two months, Richard continued to thrive on the formula Vita-Lak. When it was time for his introduction to bottled baby food, Mary gradually began to give him strained fruit, vegetables, and pureed meat. Each new variety was a trial and error situation. At first, there were some foods that he could tolerate and some he could not. Over time, he gradually began to tolerate almost all of the food she offered him.

Mary was instructed by Richard's medical team of doctors in how to administer the daily myriad of medicines to her infant son. Some of the medicines had to be given in liquid form using an eye dropper. Others needed to be crushed and the powder added to his formula. Mary was ecstatic with the results of the care she was able to provide for her son. Now that he had overcome the feeding problems he encountered at birth and was being given the mandatory medications, his overall health improved dramatically.

With a prayerful heart, Mary rejoiced as she watched Richard become a thriving baby boy. He began to develop the normal baby fat that is shown in his picture (page 11) when the family celebrated his first birthday.

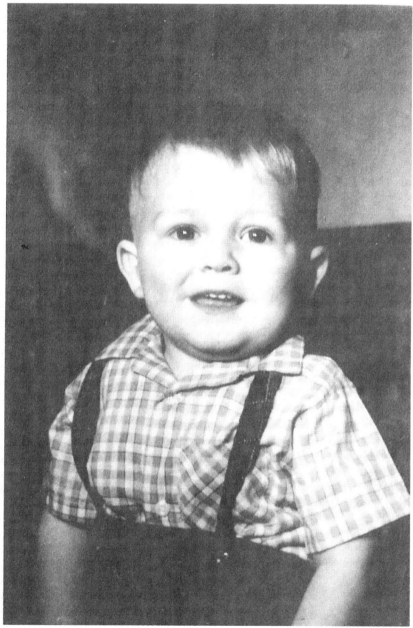

Baby Richard on his first birthday

11

Chapter 2
THE EARLY YEARS

Nine year old Daniel, four year old Ginger, and little Mitchell and Barbara helped their mother by doing light household chores. They each took turns watching their baby brother. All four of them would play and sing to entertain him until he fell asleep. Manuel was seldom home because he had to work two jobs in order to adequately support his family and pay for Richard's individual medical needs.

In spite of Mary's best efforts and with the best home care possible, before Richard's third birthday, he was in the hospital with double pneumonia four times. After each bout with pneumonia, Richard's physical activity was very limited while his weakened body slowly recovered. In order to help his labored breathing, he had to spend his nights and take his daily naps in a mist tent.

Mary was in constant contact with Richard's doctors who kept her abreast of new research being conducted, and with the latest findings for the treatment of cystic fibrosis. She read everything she could find about CF, and under the watchful eye of Richard's doctors, tried every new and suggested medication. With the help and understanding of his family, Richard endured the daily routine of being heavily medicated. Through it all he remained a cheerful, happy little boy.

With Daniel, Ginger, Mitchell and Barbara to help him along, Richard was putting whole sentences together and coloring his childhood masterpieces at an earlier age than most children. They played the usual children's games, produced beautiful pictures in their coloring books, played with Tinker Toys, Hot

Wheels, and building blocks. Consequently, this fun activity with Richard was beneficial to all of them in their physical, mental, and emotional growth.

Since Richard's siblings were older than he was, they paved the way for him to enter elementary school. He was five years old when he entered kindergarten at Highland Park Elementary School in Akron. Mary explained about the seriousness of cystic fibrosis to his very understanding and compassionate teacher. She and the school principal were amazed and very sympathetic when they learned about the large number of different medications that he had to take daily to help control the disease.

In spite of all his daily medical treatments, Richard enjoyed going to school and learning. He was a bright and highly motivated little boy, but he was physically weak. His teacher went out of her way to give Richard the special attention he needed.

Mary was nearby when Richard was asked by a playmate why he had to take so many pills every day. He answered by declaring, "I'm sick and I have to take a lot of medicines cause I've got sixty five roses."

When Mary repeated what Richard had said to the medical staff at the Cleveland Children's Hospital, they relayed the story to other families who had children with cystic fibrosis. It wasn't long afterwards that several CF support groups in Northeast Ohio were adopting the name, "Sixty Five Roses."

At the age of six, Richard entered first grade. His sister, Barbara, was just a year older than him and in the second grade. She assumed the role of "mother hen" and looked out for him all day long. During the recess periods, Ginger and Mitchell were also protective and always stayed close by him.

When Richard was approaching his seventh birthday, a new treatment was introduced that involved a physical therapy session three times a day. The new treatment would greatly reduce the danger of pneumonia.

Mary received training by the physical therapist on how to administer the new therapy. Three times a day she thumped Richard hard on his back using the heel of her hand. It took eight to ten hard thumps on his back to achieve the resultant "coughing up" of the dislodged mucus. The loosening of the mucus and the coughing up of the dislodged matter gave him intense relief from the feeling of tight congestion in his chest and kept the dreaded pneumonia at bay.

His mother, in turn, taught Manuel and Daniel how to administer the hard hand-thumping therapy. As soon as they were old enough and able to thump hard enough, she taught the technique to each of his young siblings.

To relieve the tension caused by a "have to" situation of the daily physical therapy, they began to make a game of it with much laughing and acting silly as they thumped Richard's back. The most fun for them while administering the daily thumping therapy was from creating a drum like rhythm and a sing-song cadence in time with the beats.

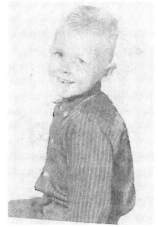 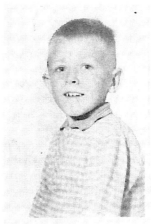

Richard, age six   *Richard, age eight*

His brothers and sisters were very supportive of Richard's needs. It never occurred to them to question the fairness of the special attention that their youngest brother received both at home and at school.

Daniel was the oldest and several grades ahead of his four younger siblings. He wasn't able to look after Richard at school, but he did more than his fair share of chores at home.

It took a lot of juggling with the clock to fit in Richard's full school day and his physical therapy treatments. Somehow the little boy realized that this was just the way life was for him. He never complained about his limited ability for rough and tumble play, and the time-consuming therapy that he had to endure.

His mother and siblings spent a lot of pleasurable time with Richard, making sure there was plenty of fun things available for him to do that kept him busy. So, instead of complaining, his ready smile and playful approach to his daily routine carried him through his full and active days.

As Richard grew older, the time-consuming special care that he required from his mother took a terrible toll on his parents and their marriage. Manuel loved his family and continued to work two jobs to support them and to earn the extra money needed for Richard's many medical needs. When Manuel did have time to spend at home, he spent it with his family. He and Richard were especially close. If he was home and it was time to administer the back-thumping physical therapy, Manuel was the one that Richard sought out to help him.

With the four younger children being so close together in age it made home life for the family difficult at best. The added time-consuming care and constant worry about CF and the possibility of Richard becoming seriously ill was always with them.

With a heavy heart and after much prayer, Mary decided she would trust in God and just do the best she could.

Mary used a written journal to record Richard's daily therapy treatments and to log in the dosages of his numerous medications. In her journal she also recorded some of his special ways of describing the world around him. Richard had a vocabulary all his own.

When speaking of the shade afforded by the window awnings, he said, "The 'yawnings' keep out the sun." If he already knew about something, he said, "I have seen that byfore."

If he didn't want to eat a particular food: "My stomach's not hungry for that."

When he joined a neighborhood peewee ball team, he explained when the ball went out of bounds: "The ball went out of bounce."

He explained his mother's one serious medical condition by telling people she had "very close" veins.

Richard would still grin when he told his young friends, "The reason I have to take a lot of medicines is 'cause I've got sixty five roses! The pills keep me from getting sick."

Richard's childhood name for cystic fibrosis has stuck. Almost fifty years later many children with CF and their families participate in a "Sixty Five Roses" support group. When strangers ask these children about their illness, they still, with an impish twinkle in their eyes, will grin and say, "I've got sixty five roses."

Richard has many happy memories about attending elementary school with his four older siblings. The children and the teachers at Highland Park School understood his physical problems and were helpful and supportive in every school activity in which he participated.

During Richard's elementary school days, Mary kept busy with her family. She also was an avid participant in community activities, including the Parent Teacher Association where she volunteered to work for the school's carnivals and other fund raising events. She was a Girl Scout and Brownies Leader, and the Den Mother for Richard's and Mitchell's Cub Scout group. She and Manuel were proud as they watched Richard and Mitchell advance to the ranks of Bear and Wolf and earn their many merit badges.

The Cystic Fibrosis Association had ninety members plus the Ohio State Women's Club. Mary and Manuel were members and she served on their board in many different capacities, including president.

At about this time, the Medina County, Ohio Cystic Fibrosis Chapter designed, published, and distributed an artful and inspirational coloring book titled, "Misty and Her Little White Cloud that Cried." The front and back covers are in vivid color and the inside artwork, designed for coloring, is beautifully done by John and Diana Delagrange.

Mary regularly took her children to church and Sunday school, and was a member of the church choir. She took all of her children to their scheduled routine doctor appointments. Richard's doctor appointments were much more often and she continued to administer his physical therapy three times a day.

She laughed and said, "My friends and family tell me I have to slow down. However, to tell the truth, I enjoy every minute of it. My husband works two jobs to make ends meet for our family and to pay for Richard's medical expenses. So we both are very busy."

Mary and Manuel were seldom able to spend time together. He would leave one job and barely have time to get to his other job. At home he could only find time to eat a hurried meal, sleep, and get out of bed to go and do the same thing over again. There was too much to do on weekends for Mary and Manuel to have the time they desperately needed with one another.

However, Manuel loved to fish. On Sunday afternoons, the one thing they could all do together was to go fishing. While Manuel and the boys fished in one of the many Akron-Canton stocked lakes and reservoirs, Mary and the girls took care of preparing the picnic fare, serving the food to the whole family, and then cleaning the area they used and packing up. Once the picnic chores were out of the way, Mary and her young daughters played games or just relaxed while Manuel and his sons fished.

Richard loved to fish. He was good at it, too. Most often he caught more fish with his cane pole, hook, line, and sinker than anyone else in the family. They used red worms and night crawlers for bait. From the time he was old enough to bait a hook, he looked forward to going fishing with his father. When for some reason they couldn't go as planned, he was always disappointed.

During the hunting seasons, other relatives took time off from work to take the boys to hunt deer, squirrel, and rabbit. Richard acquired a real love for the woods and hunting. At a very young age, he set in motion a love of the outdoors and the outdoor sports of hunting and fishing that would be with him for the rest of his life.

When his half-brother, Daniel, was twelve years old, he went to Wyoming to visit an aunt on his father's side of the family. It was only a short time after he arrived at his aunt's home that she asked Mary if Daniel could live with her. With the constant care that Richard's medical condition demanded, and caring for his three young siblings slowly wearing her down, Mary reluctantly gave her permission for Daniel to stay in Wyoming.

He was sorely missed by his brothers and sisters. Daniel's letters indicated that although he missed his family, he was very happy living with his aunt in the rugged northwest.

Mary tried her best to keep Manuel informed of all the important happenings with his children. Working two jobs made it difficult for him to be involved in their activities. With four young children and her home to care for, it wasn't possible for Mary to even consider working outside the home. She knew she would have to wait until Richard was much older to even consider finding a job.

While Richard's six years at Highland Park Elementary School gave him many good friends, beloved teachers, and still hold many happy memories for him, he describes his years at Innes Junior High as "Hell."

To begin with, there were many more children enrolled there and he had to change classes all day long. This made it physically challenging and gave him almost no time for the daily physical therapy treatments he needed. Even though Mary tried to explain to each of his new teachers about the medical problems connected with cystic fibrosis, outwardly they didn't show much, if any interest in helping him during classes.

To be fair, his mother knew that because of the large number of students in each classroom there was little chance for the teachers to give Richard the individual attention he needed. Some of the other students pestered, teased, name called, and bullied him. His teachers seemed oblivious to this and did not protect him from the oftentimes extreme cruelty of his classmates.

Because of the constant moving between classes, Richard's siblings were not able to be with him like they had been in elementary school. He was left unprotected and vulnerable. Out of the need for self preservation, he developed a "thick skin" and did not let the taunts from his classmates upset him while in school. However, although he endured their name calling and physical confrontations during the school day, remembering their taunts brought tears to his eyes when he was home and alone.

Even now, even though he is in his fifties, Richard still becomes emotionally upset with tears in his eyes when he remembers and talks about his treatment from the other children and the seemingly indifference of the teachers.

While the three years at Innes Junior High were the longest years he had ever known, the years at Kenmore High School were especially enjoyable. Richard's sister, Barbara, was one year ahead of him. She seemed to anticipate the events of each of his school days and was always nearby in case he needed anything.

Ginger and Mitchell were two or more grades ahead of him. Even so, he knew they were always nearby. Richard felt very fortunate because of the love he had from his brothers and sisters.

The memories that he has of his teachers at Kenmore High are very special to him. He said, "I'll always be grateful to them for their help and support."

Unlike the students in Innes Junior High, his classmates at Kenmore High School treated Richard with respect and went out of their way to assist him when he needed help. He made several very close, long-lasting friendships during his high school years.

All through Richard's childhood he had been shown love and support by his parents. However, Mary and Manuel faced many problems. The biggest hurdle had been financial and finding time to be alone together. Then, in 1969, when Richard was seventeen, they mutually decided to separate and later divorced.

After his parents divorced, Richard lived with his father and continued to undergo the three daily physical therapy sessions and take the large number of different medications. Manuel managed to plan his time so he could be available to administer the hard, back-thumping physical therapy. Richard managed his medications on his own. He used two boxes to keep track of his medicine. When he began, one box was filled with the thirty seven medicine bottles and the other box was empty. As he doled out each pill or capsule, he moved that bottle to the empty box. When he finished the routine, the box that had been full of medicine bottles was now empty and the empty box was now full! For fear he would get mixed up and make a mistake, no one was allowed to interrupt him in anyway until he had taken all of the medicines.

It was now 1969. Ginger was married, Mitchell was in Vietnam, and Barbara was scheduled to graduate from high school that year. Richard was on track to graduate from Kenmore High in 1970.

It was important to Richard to be financially independent. In his sophomore and junior years of high school, he had gotten needed exercise and earned tips while caddying at a nearby golf course. It was here that he developed a love for the game.

It was also during his junior year of high school that he experienced one of the most exciting and happiest days of his young life. He went to the neighborhood McDonald's Restaurant for a job interview. The restaurant manager asked him to sit down and fill out their job application form. The manager looked over his completed form and said, "Report for work at 11 o'clock tomorrow morning."

He was hired on the spot. He was ecstatic!

He worked after school and on weekends. Richard loved the newfound sense of freedom that he felt while earning his own money.

Richard excelled in every class throughout his high school experience. His sister Barbara graduated a year ahead of him and that left him pretty much on his own for his senior year. However, his teachers and school mates a Kenmore High were good to him and they gave him the educational support and special friendship that he needed.

Always in the background was the nagging worry about Richard's physical challenges from his cystic fibrosis. To see him at work, at school, participating in after school activities, and interacting with others, people had no idea the effort it took for him to achieve the resemblance of a "normal" teenager. However, it was because of his strong faith in God and a steady belief in his own abilities that he was able to achieve his goals.

When asked how he was able to do all that was required of him, with a shy smile, he explains, "My own faith in God, and the constant prayers and love of my family and friends were always with me. This helped me immensely to juggle my necessary daily CF medications and therapy treatments, school work, and my job."

One of the constants in Richard's life was his love of the outdoors. He managed to find the time, and one or two adult family members or friends with whom to go golfing and fishing. Also, he would go hunting with them during established hunting seasons. Their usual hunting grounds were in the huge Cuyahoga Valley National Park located a short distance away, northwest of Akron.

Also, he developed a love and was a dedicated fan of organized sports, including local high school competitive teams in baseball, basketball, and football. He followed closely the national standings and could quote long established statistics and record breaking achievements relative to his favorite sports figures and national teams. Richard remained an avid fan of the Cleveland

Indians, Browns, Cavaliers, and the Ohio State University Buckeyes.

His high school graduation picture (below) shows a very blond and handsome young man whose solemn demeanor reveals a person with quiet courage and a great pride in his accomplishments.

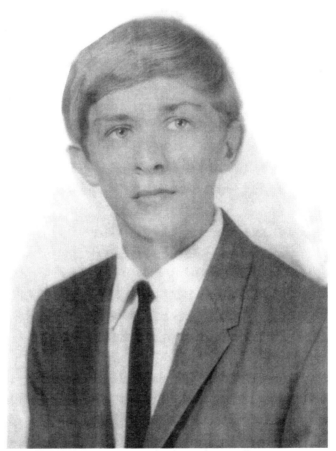

Richard's High School Graduation Picture

Chapter 3
SEEKING INDEPENDENCE

One year apart, Ginger, Mitchell, Barbara, and then Richard graduated from high school and each began their own path to becoming independent adults. All through high school Richard's plan for a higher education was to pursue a law degree from Akron University's Law School. However, his weakened body prevented him from following his dream of becoming a lawyer.

Sadly, he told his mother, "You know that going to Akron University Law School is what I've dreamed of doing, but I'm not going to begin something that I can't possibly finish."

Mary said, "Richard, with God's help, you've come a long way just by finishing high school. You've had good grades, and been an excellent student. Now, we both know you can be anything that you want to be. I agree that you don't want to set yourself up to fail. Why not continue in your job at the Coca Cola Bottling Works and see what comes along?" Richard worked at the Bottling Works in Akron. Then he took a job with a vending machine Company.

Richard had his own apartment, and for about five years he had been financially on his own. But, he was still dependent on someone in his family to administer the physical therapy three times a day. Because he wasn't happy working for someone else, he asked his parents for their opinion about what he should do. His parents talked with the rest of his family and they advised him to check around to see if there was something else, a trade, or a business that he would enjoy doing. They all assured him, "When you make up your mind as to what you want to do, you know we'll always be here for you!"

Because he wanted desperately to be financially independent, Richard had been careful to save part of his earnings over the past five years. After much prayer and discussion with his family, he decided to look into taking a local course in home appliance repair. If he completed the classes successfully, he would be eligible to take the required test to be a licensed repairman. This prospect excited him because he knew that once he was licensed, he could establish and operate his own business.

As his health permitted, he attended the home appliance repair classes and after he passed his final test, he received his license. He used his own savings to purchase the tools and equipment that he needed. And, as always, with a deep faith in God, and in himself and his abilities, he opened his own appliance repair business. Proudly, with Barbara's help he created a business card:

Whirlpool	*GE*
RICHARD C. GANNON	
KENMORE. G.E. WHIRLPOOL . HOTPOINT WASHER DRYER REPAIR	
Phone 724-1598	

Richard's charming personality, positive attitude, and an honest, sincere interest in his customers helped him to build his business. Soon, he was on a first name basis with most of his customers. He enjoyed working with his hands and skillfully repaired both large and small home appliances. From the very beginning, Richard was unusually successful. He soon had a loyal following of repeat customers who, in turn, recommended him to others and sent him all the business he could handle.

He continued to follow all of his doctors' instructions regarding the daily use of his many medications and routine physical therapy. Richard thought that his success in holding his disease at bay was because he started each day with prayer and an eagerness for tackling the day's many tasks. He told himself more than once, "There are so many things that I want to do that I don't have time to be sick!"

However, in spite of everything, he became seriously ill in 1973 and underwent surgery to remove his gall bladder. His doctors and his family were fearful that he would develop pneumonia following this surgery, but he didn't. The daily "thumping" on his back to keep the mucus loosened and the resulting coughing to expel it from his lungs had kept him free from pneumonia since he was seven years old. After the gall bladder surgery, Richard's health stabilized again for more than six years.

His daily physical therapy to keep his lungs clear had to be administered by another person. His mother and sister, Barbara, shared this daily responsibility. He and his family very carefully adhered to his medical treatment routine. Barbara and his mother checked on him constantly and because of the need for assistance in his physical therapy, he never was able to be completely independent. His family loved him and Richard knew that with his Cystic Fibrosis he would always have to be somewhat dependent on them. He did not resent this fact, but accepted it as proof of God's plan for his life which included the love of his family.

His successful home appliances repair business made it possible for Richard to realize most of his goals for independence. It wasn't long before he found a house he liked and wanted to buy. It was a small two bedroom bungalow in Firestone Park. He made an offer to the listing realty company and it was accepted. His bank approved the loan and granted him a mortgage. His spirits soared! He felt so proud! When he was able to move into his own home, the feeling that his financial independence was finally secure overwhelmed him.

His next purchase was a covered bed truck that he used for hunting and fishing. When Richard found that he had access to a boat that was large enough to use for fishing with family and friends on Lake Erie, his joy was overpowering.

Although he felt that his personal life was almost complete, his long-term plan for independence and financial freedom called for his being able to pay his mortgage and truck payments. His goal was to pay off both and be debt free as quickly as he could. Barbara often worried about Richard being able to keep up the monthly payments on his mortgage and on his truck. If his health suddenly deteriorated, it would be very hard for him to keep his home appliance repair business going. She often discussed the ominous "what if" questions with him.

When she asked him, "What will you do if you get sick and can't work? How will we manage to pay your bills?"

Richard replied, "Hey, Sis, you know that I have faith that I'll be able to keep my health under control at least until I can burn my mortgage and the note to the bank. When I finally own my home and truck, I'll be free and clear of debt. I'll truly be financially independent."

The family gave their full support to Richard and his plans. They had faith that he would be able to pay the bank loan off according to his note and contract. None of them knew how much time Richard had before the bank loan might become a problem. It was a race against time that he would be able to realize his financial goals before his cystic fibrosis interfered with his plans.

Not long after Richard bought and moved into his own house, he found a young dog that he dearly loved and who loved him in return. He named her Sheeba and the beautiful Black Labrador became his constant companion. She went everywhere with him. She kept him company while he worked at his appliance repair business. Richard, with Sheeba, also pursued his love of outdoor sports, particularly fishing and hunting.

Although Richard had fished most often at the stocked lakes and reservoirs in and around Akron and Canton, his favorite fishing place was either from a boat or around the scrubby shores of Lake Erie. Richard became quite skilled and built a reputation as an ardent fisherman. He supplied his family the year around with plenty of fish for their freezer. All he had to do was pick up his rod and reel and his tackle box, or his hunting equipment, and Sheeba was instantly "at attention," ready to go.

Richard also loved to hunt and tramp in the woods with Sheeba. Every year he impatiently waited for open season on deer. The beautiful Cuyahoga Valley National Park, located just a little northwest of Akron, was his favorite hunting grounds. It was huge, heavily wooded, had prominently laid out trails, and was overrun by a large numbers of deer.

Each year, the Park Services Administration publicly announced an invitation to all Ohio huntsmen to participate in thinning the deer population. Besides the use of his hunting rifle, Richard also became skilled in the use of the power bow. His kills provided him and his family with many delicious venison meals.

Richard was very proud of his successes and began to mount his fishing and hunting trophies on the walls of his home. Richard's family worried about his tramping around in the cold woods and about his being exposed to the dampness on the shores or on the waters of Lake Erie. They feared the cold dampness would aggravate his cystic fibrosis. And, that this might trigger a dangerous bout with pneumonia. However, in the long run, they felt that the therapeutic benefit of doing the things he really loved far outweighed the possible health dangers he might encounter.

Over the years, Richard had remained close to his father. Manuel had remarried and made a new life for himself with a new family. After the years of being a single mom, Mary's life, too, was about to change forever. In 1972 Mary met Charles Moon. They fell in love and made plans to be married right away.

After Mary and Charles were settled into their marriage, and with her children grown and on their own, Mary decided she wanted to find a job where she could work with children. In 1973 she began working for Summit County Children Services in Akron Ohio. She held the position of child care worker, or house parent, at Anderson Village. Anderson Village was the agency's twenty-four-hour residential facility for dependent, abused, and neglected children who were in the legal custody of Summit County.

Mary was in charge of a residential unit, or cottage, that housed up to twelve children. She provided the nurturing care for each child that ideally would have been provided in a caring home with their natural, or biological, parents. To the children for whom Mary provided twenty-four-hour residential care, she was simply "Mom Moon."

Because of her work schedule as a live-in child care worker, Mary was hard pressed to find the time she needed to help with Richard's physical therapy. This fell more and more on Barbara's shoulders. Barb, too, became employed at Summit County Children Services as the Administrative Assistant to the agency's Finance Director. When her mother wasn't available to provide the physical therapy, she stopped at Richard's home before work in the morning, again at noon, and on her way home from work in the evening. Richard managed very well on his own in taking his many medications throughout the day, but he was totally dependent, three times a day, on another person for the physical therapy.

With a lot of prayer and complete trust in God, he and his family were still able to assume the extra burden that was necessary in order to care for a person with cystic fibrosis.

As the years passed, Richard's business remained successful and he was able to become financially independent. Always in the back of his mind was one big worry, a nagging fear, "Will my health problems with Cystic Fibrosis get in the way of my goals?"

However, Richard's faith was enduring. He was comfortable enough with his lifelong personal relationship with God that he spoke boldly in prayer, saying, "I trust You, Lord, to provide a way for me. If it is Your will, my health will improve. Whatever is Your will, I'll accept it. I thank You, God, for my family. Lord, please take care of them and bless them. I believe that I will live. I couldn't say this if I didn't have Your abiding love and the love of my family. You will prevail in my life. I know, Lord, that You will always take care of me."

Richard's health continued to allow him to live close to a normal life. He was careful, never missed taking his medications and having someone help him with his physical therapy. In 1978, when he was twenty four years old he met a lovely young woman named Sandy. They fell in love.

After a lot of soul searching and doubts about the wisdom of getting married because of the seriousness of his health problems, Richard asked for guidance from God as to what he should do. He loved Sandy and because of his deep feelings for her, he did not want to become a burden to her. He decided he would trust God to lead him and then he took a "leap of faith." He asked Sandy to be his wife. She said "Yes."

Richard had never been happier. He and Sandy were married when he was twenty five. They set up housekeeping in Richard's house and for a time were very happy together. However, after just one year it was apparent that they were no longer the happy couple they once had been. Sadly, the union of Richard and Sandy did not last. When Richard was twenty six, by mutual agreement, he and Sandy were divorced.

Although he was devastated, Richard accepted the separation and divorce as God's will. After a sorrowful period of mourning the loss of what might have been, he was able to adjust to losing Sandy and was able to go on with his life.

The reality of the situation was that with his health problems, he realized that God's plan for him did not include a lasting marriage. He was afraid he had been selfish and had not taken into account that God had a life plan for Sandy, too. When the divorce was final, she, too, was able to go on with her life.

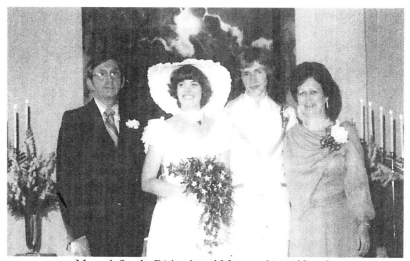

Manuel, Sandy, Richard, and Mary on his wedding day

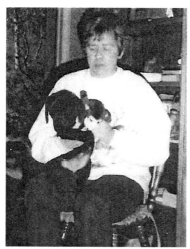

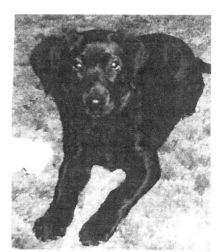

Richard's puppy, Sheeba   *Sheeba, Richard's constant companion*

Chapter 4
HORRENDOUS HEALTH CHALLENGES

With the constant support of his loving family, Richard continued to live as normal a life as possible. He carefully followed his daily routine of physical therapy and medications. Although rarely, he still had life threatening bouts with pneumonia. Usually, he would have advance warning when pneumonia threatened him and could go to the Rainbow Babies and Adults Medical Center in Cleveland. However, there were times that the high fever and pain would strike without warning and his family would rush him to the Cleveland Medical Facility. When he was well enough, he would return home to recuperate.

His home appliance repair business provided him with an adequate income. With Sheeba as his constant companion over the years, he was able to pursue his love of outdoor sports. With family and friends, he fished in the well stocked Akron area lakes and reservoirs as well as on Lake Erie. He hiked the nature trails and hunted, in season, in the Cuyahoga Valley National Park.

Beginning in 1988, Richard developed diabetes that required him, in addition to his other myriad of daily medications, to add enzymes. He also had to have four injections of insulin a day. His doctors informed him that this was a sign that his body was breaking down.

It was in November 1990, that Richard became very ill. This illness wasn't the forerunner of pneumonia. He quickly became severely jaundiced and was admitted to the Intensive Care Unit at the University Hospitals of Cleveland. After a battery of tests, and exploratory surgeries, the doctors informed Richard and his family that, in order for him to live, he needed a liver transplant. Then almost immediately they changed their prognosis to include additional organ transplants. They would place Richard on the waiting list to receive a triple organ transplant: a liver, a kidney, and a pancreas.

Because of a long organ donor waiting list for other patients, this promised to be a terrifyingly long vigil. However, Richard was so close to death that his name was moved to the top of the donor waiting list. Also, because his condition was life threatening, he remained in the Intensive Care Unit. But, his family was allowed to visit with him much more frequently and remain longer than the usual twenty minutes each day.

While waiting for a donor, Richard's liver failed and his body became even more acutely jaundiced. His family and friends placed Richard's name on many prayer lists and waited.

There was glad rejoicing when their prayers were finally answered. A suitable donor was found and the sixteen-hour triple organ transplant surgery was performed on January 10, 1991.

It was later learned that the donor organs came from a grieving family whose son had been declared "brain dead." Their son had expressed wishes to be an organ donor if the need should arise. Tests showed him to be a match to Richard. His parents gave their permission for their son's organs to be donated and this selfless act saved Richard's life.

Mary stated, "My family and I will be forever grateful to the unknown parents who made the decision to donate their son's organs. Their son saved our son's life. God bless them!"

The University Hospitals of Cleveland reported that this was the first time that one patient had received a triple organ transplant. The news of this medical marvel literally went around the world.

An article written by Michael Drexler, Plain Dealer Reporter, April 25, 1991, was as follows:

"TRIPLE TRANSPLANT A MIRACLE"
"RICHARD C. GANNON, CANAL FULTON, (Ohio) BATTLED A NIGHTMARE FOR MONTHS."

"Gannon was a prisoner, bound to a hospital bed, unable to move. He tried to escape, but to no avail. He struggled and struggled…and then woke up in a cold sweat. He asked himself in the white glare of a hospital room: 'Will I ever get out? Will I live?'

The answer was 'Yes.'

Gannon smiled all the way home March 28 after a triple organ transplant – pancreas, liver, and kidneys – the first triple transplant in Ohio, performed at University Hospitals. According to a spokesman for the United Network for Organ Sharing, which is responsible for organ matches nationwide, the procedure was among 'only a handful' ever done in the United States.

'This is extremely rare,' said Alissa Frietag, a spokesman for the Ohio Solid Organ Transplant Consortium, which represents the seven Ohio hospitals that can perform extra-renal (other than kidney) transplants.

Gannon, 38, who has Cystic Fibrosis and diabetes, said he felt 'awful' before the surgery, but the only thing that bothers him now is his left leg. It's a little swollen. 'That's it,' he said.

His doctor said if Gannon hadn't had the transplant operation, he would have died.

Gannon, who has been home for four weeks, said yesterday: 'I feel like a new man. It's amazing what they can do these days. One of my doctors's told me I might be one of the few people in the world with these three organs transplanted. I had no idea all this was going to happen to me.'

Dr. James A. Schulak, director of transplantation at University Hospitals, is no less amazed at the outcome. He was part of the three-member surgery team that performed the 16-hour operation January 10.

'This is an Ohio and a Cleveland first, and it went very well,' Schulak said, noting that the combination of organs and the fact that Gannon has Cystic Fibrosis made the operation even more unusual. 'It was extremely gratifying to be able to have a patient with so many debilities feeling better than he has in a long time.'

Cystic Fibrosis is an inherited disease that affects many of the body's organs and leads to their eventual destruction. Most people who have Cystic Fibrosis do not live past childhood. In Gannon's case, the disease affected his liver, pancreas and kidneys.

His kidney failure was secondary to his other illnesses. Schulak said he had checked around the country with other transplant surgeons, and 'No one had ever heard of this before.'

Before the operation, Gannon had to inject insulin four times a day. He also took enzymes and many other medications. His liver problems presented the most lethal threat.

Gannon was deemed a good bet for such a risky operation because of his emotional strength. Schulak said a good candidate for transplant surgery must 'fully appreciate the gravity of their transplant. And it is important for them to be a compliant patient. In his case, there was no problem. He had an excellent mental attitude. He has demonstrated that by living 38 years with Cystic Fibrosis. He is a winner, and we felt very good about that right off the bat.'

Gannon, a self employed appliance repairman before he became seriously ill, had the transplants in the nick of time. He entered the hospital November 15 with abdominal pain and nausea. The day he signed in, Gannon thought he was just having some minor lung problems due to his Cystic Fibrosis and had planned to get some deer hunting in before season's end.

But he got sicker. As his condition became critical, his doctors decided to research the possibility of a liver transplant. Further study brought the possibility of a triple transplant. Schulak and his team believed that replacing Gannon's diseased liver, pancreas and kidneys would cure most of the conditions caused by his Cystic Fibrosis, including the diabetes.

The transplant would provide no cure for Cystic Fibrosis, which has no known cure, but it might extend Gannon's life, Schulak believed.

Gannon's unusual candidacy was reviewed by the Ohio Solid Organ Transplant Consortium, which reviews all transplants in Ohio, and was approved in mid-December.

Three University Hospital transplant surgeons-Doctors James T. Mayes, Kent H. Johnston, and Schulak performed as the surgical equivalent of a 'tag team,' trading places and taking short breaks during the long operation. Nothing went wrong (during the surgery). Gannon awoke to find himself in great pain but with renewed hope.

Gannon, like many transplant patients, suffered pneumonia after the surgery, and went into a week-long coma from a slight stroke. Then he bounced back, though he remained in intensive care for a month.

During that time, Gannon recalled, the nightmares dominated every night of sleep.

'I'd wake up from them and I didn't know if I was sleeping or dreaming. I'd dream that I was in a prison, and I wanted to escape. I kept trying, but they tied me down to the bed. I still tried to get out, and I was hanging onto the side of the bed,' Gannon remembered. 'During that time, I was in a lot of pain and I was in intensive care for a month.'

After his bout with pneumonia, the stroke and months of terrible pain, Gannon turned the corner. He started eating foods such as chocolate and peanuts- things he hadn't been able to eat in years.

Then, with the help of a cane, he started walking. At home with his sister Ginger Pedani, he spends his days in mild ecstasy over what he calls 'a miracle.'

The total bill for the operation was $450,000, which was paid for by Medicaid, Medicare and the Ohio State Bureau of Children with Medical Handicaps, a state program that helps children and eligible adults who have medical disabilities. Gannon qualified for the program because no insurance company would sell him health insurance.

Gannon said perhaps the nicest thing that happened through all his struggles was seeing his brother, Mitchell, who was allowed by the Air Force to come back from Saudi Arabia during the Persian Gulf War to see him.

The war soon came to an end. 'My brother was here for two weeks. It was a real surprise. I'm still emotional about it,' Gannon said, his voice breaking. 'That really helped me. The doctor said it was real important that I have family support. I wouldn't have made it without them.

I don't take anything for granted anymore,' Gannon said. 'I really value my life. I thank the people who donated the organs for me. I thank God, my family, the transplant team, the hospital staff–everyone. Now, I love life."

Richard and his family publicly expressed their deep appreciation to the Bureau for Children with Medical Handicaps (BCMH) for their unlimited support for Richard during his long hospital stay and through all the struggles with physical therapy and rehabilitation.

The Mission Statement of the Agency:

"The mission of the Bureau for children with medical handicaps is to assure, through the development and support of high quality coordinated systems, that children with special health care needs and their families obtain comprehensive care and services which are family-centered, community-based and culturally competent."

Direct health care services include and are defined as follows:
"The Bureau for Children's services is generally delivered between a health professional and a patient in an office, clinic, or emergency room. For example, well-child care visit; visit to a doctor for an acute health care condition; follow-up visit to a specialist for a chronic condition, physical therapy, occupational therapy, respiratory therapy, inpatient and outpatient medical services, allied health services, lab, and etc."
The age eligibility criteria that assured Richard of financial assistance for his high medical

costs were that children were covered from birth to 21 years of age; except for individuals with Cystic Fibrosis for whom there is no age limit.

Right after the triple organ transplant surgery, Richard said he had all kinds of serious problems, including the inevitable pneumonia, a brain infection, a stroke, and was in a coma for six days.

However, Richard told Barbara, "God was with me all the way through this, and I had faith that I wasn't going to die. Ever since I can remember, I have felt that God has a life plan for me. I didn't feel that I had completed God's plan for me, yet."

Richard's successful experience under the care of the skillful team of surgeons who performed his triple organ transplant in January, 1991, paved the way for additional advances in treatment of Cystic Fibrosis. In 1993-94, a team of doctors, including some of those involved with the triple organ transplant surgery for Richard co-authored a remarkable landmark medical journal paper titled:

"Restoration of Exocrine Pancreatic Function Following a Pancreas-liver-kidney
Transplantation in a Cystic Fibrosis Patient."   *(Munksgaard---*
1994 printed in Denmark-
ISSN 0902-0063)

The doctors cited in the article are Robert C. Stern, James T. Mayes, Fredrick L. Weber, Jr., Edmond W. Blades, and James

A. Schulak. (See photographs, below, of Richard and some of his doctors)

The medical facilities cited in the article are the Department of Pediatrics, Surgery and Medicine, Case Western Reserve University School of Medicine, University Hospitals of Cleveland, and Rainbow Babies and Children's Hospital, Cleveland, Ohio, U.S.A.

Also reported in this article was information about grant support for ongoing research and treatment programs that is provided by the National Institutes of Health and by grants from the Cystic Fibrosis Foundation and United Way of Greater Cleveland.

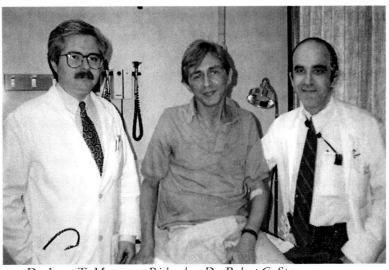

Dr. James T. Mayes   Richard   Dr. Robert C. Stern

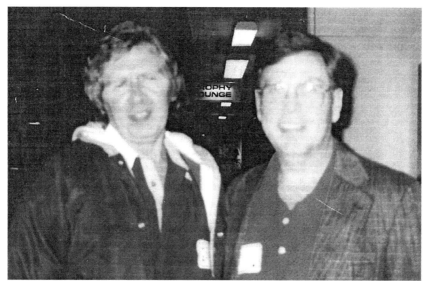

Richard and Dr. James A. Schulak

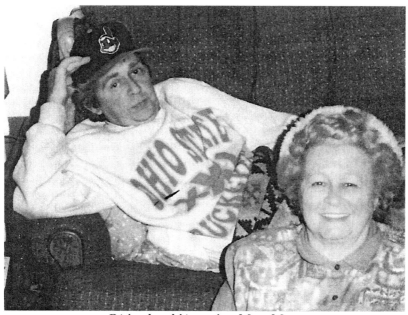

Richard and his mother, Mary Moon
(Recuperating at sister's (Ginger) home in Canal Fulton)

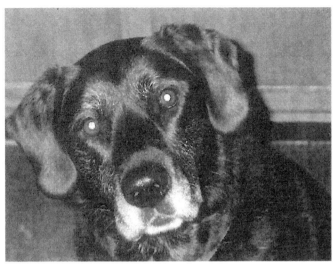
Sheeba – growing older

Richard entered Cleveland University Hospital on November 15, 1990 and was not released until March 28, 1991. After his release from the hospital in Cleveland, he went to the Edwin Shaw Hospital in Akron for several months of rehabilitation. It was about three months before he could walk again.

All in all, Richard made a positive recovery from his triple organ transplant surgery. His long stay in the Cleveland medical facilities was followed by the additional months in rehabilitation at Edwin Shaw. He still needed more recuperative time and was spending it in Canal Fulton with his sister, Ginger Pedani, who is an R.N. It was here that Richard discovered he had an even deeper personal conviction that God was a profound entity in his life. He attended his sister's church in Canal Fulton. It was during one of these church services that Richard re-dedicated and totally surrendered his life to God. He was convinced that part of God's plan for him was the 'call' he urgently felt to advocate for CF patients and their families.

In fulfillment of this call, Richard became a sought-after public speaker. His presentations included his personal experiences while living with cystic fibrosis, his abiding faith in God and the awesome power of prayer, and the love and support he received from family and friends.

He spoke to many different organizations, including The Kent State Nursing Class and several of the Northeast Ohio Sixty Five Roses CF Support Groups. His presentations were always inspirational in describing his lifelong coping with cystic fibrosis, the symptoms, the care, and what can be done to help other CF patients.

He described the circumstances leading up to his triple-organ transplant and the sixteen-hour surgery. He told of how the medical skills of his doctors had saved his life, and he paid tribute to the professional commitment and loving care he had received from the University Hospitals of Cleveland, his dedicated nurses and other staff. He found it hard to not become emotional when he described the selflessness of the loving parents who donated their son's organs so that he might live.

Richard declared how the love and prayers of his family and friends had made such an awesome difference in his life. When talking with a group, he always displayed an up-beat attitude. Richard was a special inspiration to families who had a loved one with cystic fibrosis and to those who were, themselves, personally coping with the disease.

In September, 1993, the International Office of Transplant Recipients International Organization (TRIO) held its Fifth Annual Conference at the Renaissance Hotel, in Washington,

D.C. The theme for their annual meeting was, "Meeting the Challenge: Awareness, Advocacy and Education."

The invited honorees included:
- Vice President Al Gore to receive the Starzl Award
- Senator Strom Thurmond (R-SC) and his family to present the Organ Donor Family Award
- Secretary of Health and Human Services, Donna Shalala
- Organ Donor Families
- Organ Transplant Recipients

One of the most moving activities of the entire meeting was the "Tree Of Life" ceremony. Each organ transplant recipient was asked to prepare a meaningful memento so that they could take part in the ceremony by placing that personal token on the "Tree of Life."

The following is from the article in "Lifelines Lite" written by Joyce Willig, TRIO Board member:

"As each recipient approaches the Tree of Life bearing his or her special token, that gift becomes both a personal affirmation of the bond between donor and recipient- as well as a validation of the sanctity of the human spirit."

The number of attendees at the TRIO Fifth Annual Conference in Washington D.C., including the high ranking public officials, that was coupled with a demonstrated high degree of sincere emotional support for all CF victims and their families was very impressive. Also, the same high degree of respect that was extended to the CF transplant recipients and their families, and the families of the transplant donors left a lasting impression on Richard, his mother and sister, Barbara.

To celebrate Richard's fortieth birthday, his family organized a "Roast" party for him. The following is the written remarks from his next door neighbor and good friend, Ronald Rush, Akron:

A TRIBUTE TO RICK GANNON

A few thoughts about our very good friend and next door neighbor, Rick Gannon:

Rick is a very generous person. If all of the fish that he's given to us over the years were laid end-to-end in a straight line, starting from his house, EPA officials and animal-rights radicals from four counties would be beating down his door.

His fish supplies us with many important vitamins and minerals-including mercury! Whenever it gets too hot I send Pat outside so she doesn't screw the ceiling up (She smokes continuously).

Rick has also given us much deer meat. Incidentally, Rick never shoots a deer unless he's assured that he'll get to chase it first into the next time zone! He gets so much exercise that way that he doesn't have to lift a finger for the next eleven months.

Happy birthday, Rick, You're one of the good ones, pal. God bless you.

Ron & Pat   9/19/92 at 12:16 PM

(This is just one of the many "Roasts" to Richard by family and friends at the party celebrating his 40th)

Over the next few years, Richard had so many more surgeries that his mother called him her "bionic son" after the television series "The Six Million Dollar Man." Richard and his family believe he is the only living cystic fibrosis patient who has had so many different organ transplants and surgeries.

In January 1991 Richard had the Triple Organ Transplant. Then, he had the following additional surgeries: In 1995 a knee replacement; in 1997 a shoulder replacement; in November, 1998 another shoulder replacement and a second kidney transplant; and in 2001 a second knee replacement

Then, he was admitted to Cleveland University Hospital in April 2001 for surgery to correct sleep apnea. Half way through the surgery, he started bleeding excessively. The surgical procedure was discontinued and has not been rescheduled.

On his fiftieth birthday, September 19 2002, Richard's sister, Barb, sent an e-mail to his many friends that gave the following update on his activities:

"Richard enjoyed a summer of fishing and taking care of his dog, Sheeba, and his yard. He is scheduled for a hip replacement in December. So keep him in your prayers. Thanks for all your help in making his birthday an unforgettable one!"

Richard continued his daily battle against cystic fibrosis. He is living proof of what a person faced with overwhelming odds can accomplish. He readily admits that he was never alone. He had his deep faith in God's abiding love, faith in his own abilities, skillful doctors, and the love and prayers of family and friends.

Barb believed and often said, "Never sell short the power of the human spirit. My brother has proven over and over that when one refuses to give up or give in to overpowering adverse life circumstances, that anything is possible with God to those who trust and believe in Him."

Chapter Five
ONGOING MEDICAL RESEARCH AND TECHNOLOGICAL ADVANCES

Richard and his family tried to keep abreast of the latest research, laboratory testing, and approved treatments available for patients with cystic fibrosis. A recorded chronological history of the progress being made by medical science shows that the treatment of cystic fibrosis is improving almost daily. The following is from an article by Tim Friend in USA Today, dated Tuesday, April 14, 1998 (Page 7D).

"Treatment of Cystic Fibrosis on the fast track"

"13 pills three times a day…Eric Kast, of Norman Oklahoma, swallows them with pride. He believes he is contributing to an eventual cure for Cystic Fibrosis.

CF is the most common fatal, inherited disease among whites, affecting 30,000 children and young adults in the USA. Most will die from lung damage caused by the buildup of thick mucus and chronic infections.

But progress in treating this fatal disease is accelerating at a remarkable pace. When Kast was born in 1968, median life expectancy was just over 10 years. By 1980, with improved medical care, boys and girls could expect to go to high school and were living to age eighteen.

Then scientists began unlocking the secrets of the physiology, and fundamental discoveries in the basic sciences began streaming out of laboratories like smoke from a genie's bottle.

By 1989, Kast and others with CF could not only expect to go to college, they also had time to marry and start a family. Life expectancy jumped to 29. The same year, a gene mutation responsible for 90% of cases was found, and the genie was out of the bottle for good.

Since then, the gene has been giving up its secrets as quickly as scientists can tease them out. And the findings have been rapidly transferred to studies involving CF patients. Kast has been among the first to join experimental trials and to benefit from advances when they are made.

The mound of pills Kast has been taking is for a study of an experimental drug called phenylbutyrate. It is one of several new drugs that, next to gene therapy, represent the most remarkable potential advance yet in cystic fibrosis.

Phenylbutyrate, a second drug called CPX, and a third, Duramycin, are designed specifically to repair the molecular havoc created by a gene mutation that is locked in the cells that line Kast's lungs and airways.

Before discovery of the gene and the ensuing study of the mutation, scientists could not have conceived of developing such highly targeted drugs. Today, this approach, which integrates basic science with gene discovery, represents the way most drugs will be created in the new millennium.

'We are now able to create designer drugs based on the detailed molecular biology of a disease,' says Francis Collins, Director, National Institute, at the National Institutes of Health in Bethesda, Maryland. 'And we are in fact coming up with drugs that we would never have been able to think of before.'

Collins and his research team discovered the Cystic Fibrosis gene while at the University of Michigan. Lap-Chee Tsui and John Riordam discovered the gene at the same time at their lab at the University of Toronto. The Cystic Fibrosis Foundation, in Bethesda, credits all three with the discovery.

'Since discovery of the gene, I've been given hope for the future,' Kast says. 'In addition to the gene therapy, they have many drugs that they are developing. That gives us hope that if one doesn't work, another one will.'

The article went on to explain:

Understanding behavior of the CF gene:

Scientists have rapidly expanded their study of Cystic Fibrosis since the 1989 discovery of the gene that causes the disease. More than 12,000 scientific papers have been published as of April, 1998. 'Most of these focus on understanding the behavior of the gene and its protein, understanding chloride channels and testing new drug therapies.' Says

Robert J. Beall, President and CEO of the Cystic Fibrosis Foundation……

Tracking the progress:

- 1990 Scientists make a normal copy of the Cystic Fibrosis transmembrane conductance regulator (CFTR) gene and correct CF cells in the lab. Gene therapy becomes a possibility.
- 1992 Researchers create a mouse model for CF, providing a reliable way to test gene and drug therapies. They also learn how to make large amounts of CFTR protein and begin learning to create protein-targeted therapies.
- 1993 The first human gene therapy studies begin at three sites. University of Iowa researchers report that CF cells in their human patients were corrected. The Food and Drug Administration approves the first drug for CF in 30 years. It is Pulmozyme and is designed to break up thick mucus in the lungs.
- 1994 Two gene therapy trials begin, and studies begin with the first patients treated.
- 1995 A four-year clinical trial of ibuprofen shows that high doses under controlled conditions can reduce lung inflammation in CF patients. And
- The first aerosol gene therapy trials begin. Until now, gene therapy trials have used modified cold viruses to deliver genes. The University of Alabama becomes the first to test microscopic beads called liposomes that contain genes. Johns Hopkins University tests a new delivery system called adeno-associated virus.

- 1996 University of Iowa researchers discover the underlying reason people with CF are so receptive to bacterial infections: Apparently because of high salt concentrations outside cells, a naturally occurring substance that wards off infection is unable to perform its job.
- 1997 CPX is approved for studies. University of Pennsylvania researchers discover a molecule called HHBD-1 that may be a key link between CF cells and fatal lung infections. And
- The University of Washington-Seattle and Patho-Genesis Corporation begin mapping and sequencing the entire genome of Pseudomonas aeruginosa, which is the main bug that infects CF patients' lungs. This will provide new treatment approaches. And
- The FDA approves TOBI, an inhaled antibiotic that has been shown to improve lung function and reduce the number of days that patients spend in hospitals.
- 1998 Researchers finish phenylbutyrate trials. The Cystic Fibrosis Foundation begins a partnership with biotechnology companies to provide money for further development of drugs."

An article in the Washington Post by Staff Writer William Booth was headlined "Test Identifies Carriers of Cystic Fibrosis – Routine Screening of Couples Possible," and reads:

"Medical researchers have developed a new genetic test that can spot three-quarters of all adults who risk having children with cystic fibrosis, raising the possibility that many couples will undergo routine screening and that fetuses that carry the defective gene could be aborted."

The article went on to quote Doctor Harvey Colton, who cautioned the extended use of the newly developed genetic tool.

"Colton and other researchers question whether aborting a fetus that carries the defective gene is justified, when new therapies could be soon developed to extend the quality and span of life for those with cystic fibrosis into their 40s and 50s."

"I would argue vigorously against mandatory testing," Colton said.

The new laboratory tests follow by six months the announcement by Canadian and American researchers that they finally had found the gene that causes Cystic Fibrosis.

Chapter Six
MEMORIES AND MEMENTOS

The following poem was written by Richard's Mother, Mary. She said she was inspired to write it because of how bravely her son faced his illness and coped with its limitations on his life.

THINK POSITIVE
By Mary Elizabeth Moon

When the pressures of life are too great,
Walk away from that prison of hate,
Give your family their space,
And you need yours.
Your love for them will continue to grow.
And theirs for you, somehow we just know,

We need to turn to those who love us,
Our family, our friends,
And God above us,
Who always give us strength to carry on.

Being depressed is just a state of mind,
Think positive! Be happy!
And then you will find,
There is so much love in this world,
When we seek it.
And when with our loved ones whom we know,
We will always have love and keep it,
So, let go of the past,

Rejoice to the World,
I'm happy! I'm happy!
I'm happy at last!

Mary locked away in her heart many precious memories.
She gathered and treasured the special mementos that
documented the love and support that Richard received from his
family and friends.

One of the most treasured is the following poem that was
written by Richard's Aunt Naomi Faye Stevens.

THE GREAT ARTIST OF SPRING FLOWERS
By Naomi Faye Stevens
(For my Nephew, Richard C. Gannon)

As the beautiful spring flowers start to peep through
the dark earthly ground,
They start to spread their fragrance all around;
A sneak preview of another spring season,
Alluring colorful and beauty;
And for a special reason.

As God paints them with his brush of nature,
A bonanza of fantastic colors to enjoy for,
Every woman, man, girl, and boy;
And for the whole world to share,
That he put in our tender care.

Then the wild flowers of the field will
Begin to sway and sing,
As God fans them with his angel wings;

Celebrating a new artistic year,
Of beautiful spring flowers.

A touch of God's nature all bundled into one;
What beauty and happiness they will bring,
In the spring seasons and in the wind;
The echoes of the world's flowers,
Will rapture and live to bloom again.

The following letter was written and distributed in 1990 by The Partnership for Organ Donation and Transplant Recipients International Organization (TRIO)
At that time their addresses were:

The Partnership for Organ Donation
2 Oliver Street
Boston, MA 02109

TRIO
244 N. Bellefield Avenue
Pittsburgh, PA 15213

A DIFFERENT KIND OF LOVE LETTER

Dear Friend,
Some people might call this a chain letter, but we like to think of it as a love letter. It is a different kind of love letter. It was started by a group of transplant recipients and, with your help we hope that it will travel throughout the country encouraging people to discuss their wishes about organ and tissue donation with their families.

Did you know that you have the power to save up to six lives? If you choose to become an organ donor, it's possible for you to do just that. But what you need to do first is inform your family of your intentions.

Of course, organ donation happens only after you have died, and your family will be called upon to make a decision. You can make that moment easier for them by communicating your decision in advance.

And you can help people awaiting a transplant to enjoy life again through your gift of love and life.

Consider these facts:

- In 1993, 18,000 lives were saved or enhanced as a result of organ transplants.
- 85% of Americans support organ donation.
- More than 33,000 Americans are currently awaiting an organ transplant.
- Nine people will die today without receiving the life-saving organs they need.

Don't wait until it's too late. Even if you have a signed donor card or driver's license, talk to your family about becoming an organ donor. Then copy this letter and send it on to five friends. If you have a personal connection to donation or transplantation, we encourage you to share your story along with this letter. You can truly give others a second chance at life.

For those in the Cleveland area who wish to donate organs of their loved ones, please contact:

LifeBanc
Tower East Office Building
20600 Chagrin Blvd. Suite 350
Cleveland, OH 44122-5343

TO REMEMBER ME
By Robert N. Test

The day will come when my body will be upon a white sheet
Neatly tucked under four corners of a mattress, located in a
Hospital busily occupied with the living and the dying.
At a certain moment, a doctor will determine that my brain has
ceased to function, and that, for all intents and purposes, my life
has stopped.

When that happens, do not attempt to instill artificial life into my
body by the use of a machine, and don't call this my death bed.
Let it be called the "Bed of Life."
And let my body be taken from it to help
Others lead fuller lives.

Give my sight to the man, who has never seen a sunrise,
A baby's face or love in the eyes of a woman.
Give my heart to a person whose own heart has caused
Nothing but endless days of pain.

Give my blood to the teen-ager who was pulled from
The wreckage of his car
So that he might live to see his grandchildren play.
Give my kidneys to one who depends on a machine
To exist from week to week.

Take my bones, every muscle, every fiber and nerve
In my body, and find a way to make a crippled child walk.
Explore every corner of my brain. Take my cells, if necessary,
And let them grow, so that some day,

SIXTY FIVE ROSES: THE RICHARD GANNON STORY

BOGGS-QUALLS

A speechless boy will shout at the crack of a bat.
And a deaf girl will hear the sound of rain against her window.

Burn what is left of me and scatter the ashes to the winds, to help
the flowers grow.
If you must bury something, let it be my faults,
My weaknesses, and all prejudice against my fellow man.

Give my sins to the devil,
Give my soul to God.
If by chance, you wish to remember me,
Do it with a kind deed or word to someone who needs you.

If you do all I have asked, I will live forever.

MAKE A MIRACLE-----BE AN EYE AND ORGAN DONOR

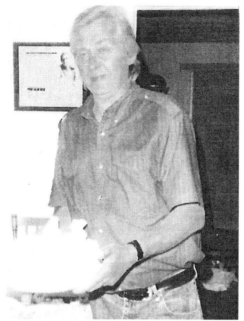

Richard's Birthday Party - 1997

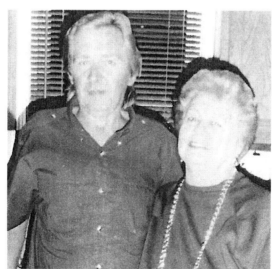

Richard and Mother, Mary Moon, 2000

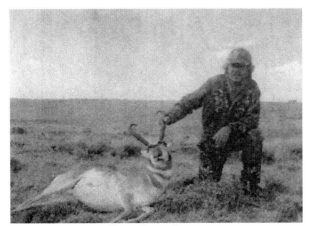

Deer Open Season

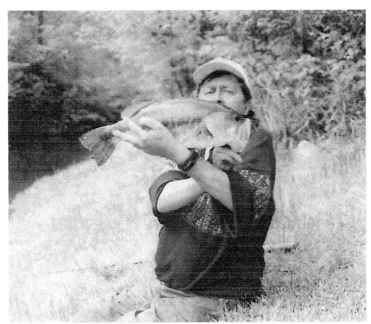

Akron/Canton Area Fishing Waters
Richard's Catch Of The Day

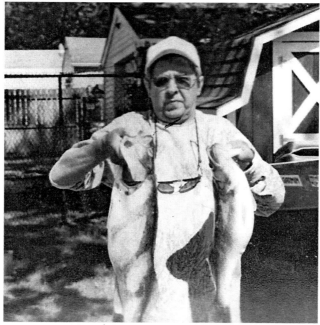

Akron/Canton Area Fishing Waters

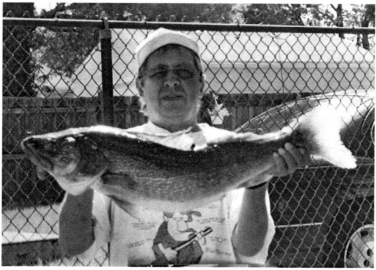

Lake Erie Fishing

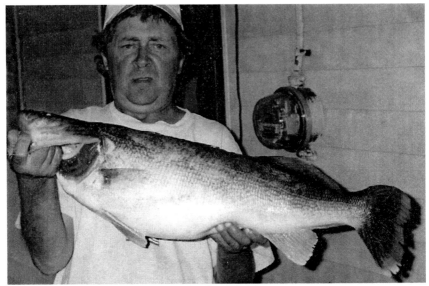

Lake Erie Fishing

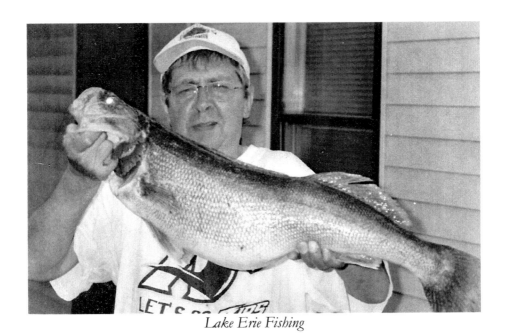

Lake Erie Fishing

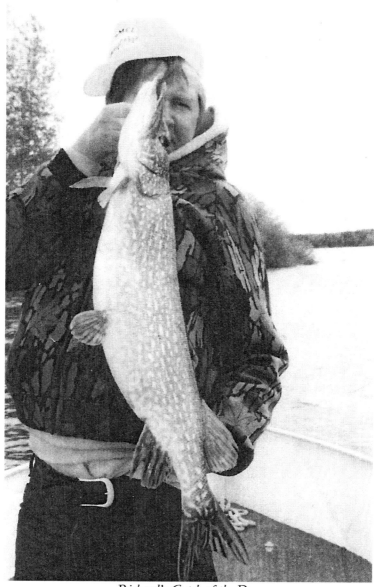

Richard's Catch of the Day
Lake Erie

EPILOGUE

As living proof that he is, indeed, one of life's survivors, Richard lived a full and active life well into his fifties. Sadly, he passed away on March 25, 2007. All of his life he demonstrated great courage, an unfaltering faith in God, and the awesome power of prayer. His shy, but optimistic, ready smile, and easy going personality was and is an inspiration to the rest of us who must meet our own life challenges every day.

Richard's obituary, provided by his sister, Barbara Brunk, to The Cleveland Plain Dealer echoed the inspirational accomplishments of his life:

"RICHARD CUMMINS GANNON

The inspirational life of Richard Cummins Gannon came to a peaceful end on March 25, 2007, at the age of 54. Born on September 19, 1952 with Cystic Fibrosis and given just a few years to live, Richard defied all odds. He was a 1970 graduate of Kenmore High School and later completed appliance repair school, allowing him to start his own business. The AARCEE Washer Dryer Repair Service, which he successfully ran for 12 years.

He was also an avid fisherman and hunter, and devotedly followed "his" area sports teams. These included the local college team and the major leagues of the Cavs, Indians, Browns, and, of course, the Ohio State Buckeyes.

Richard will be best remembered, however, for making medical history in 1991. His health failing, he became the first individual in the state of Ohio to successfully receive a triple-organ transplant (kidney, pancreas and liver). To this day, he remains an inspiration to all who knew him for his incredible determination and will.

The family would like to offer special thanks to so many who were instrumental in the success story of Richard. First, our thanks go to Doctor Robert C. Stern, Jr. who lovingly cared for him over the last 42 years. And secondly, to the 7th floor Adult CF Division at Rainbow Babies and Children's Hospital for their endless dedication and care.

Also, the family is forever grateful to Dr. James Schulak and staff and Dr. Anthony Post and staff of the University Hospitals Transplant Division, for their medical breakthrough in 1991, and to LifeBanc, for making the impossible possible."

Among the family survivors listed in the obituary is his grandmother, Lorene Gannon (101 years old) of Ironton, Ohio.

Printed in the United States
202332BV00007B/1-105/P